Adama Noumou Doumbia

OCULAR COMPLICATIONS AND DAMAGE IN HEMODIALYSIS PATIENTS

Adama Noumou Doumbia

OCULAR COMPLICATIONS AND DAMAGE IN HEMODIALYSIS PATIENTS

EYE DISORDERS IN HEMODIALYSIS PATIENTS

ScienciaScripts

Imprint

Any brand names and product names mentioned in this book are subject to trademark, brand or patent protection and are trademarks or registered trademarks of their respective holders. The use of brand names, product names, common names, trade names, product descriptions etc. even without a particular marking in this work is in no way to be construed to mean that such names may be regarded as unrestricted in respect of trademark and brand protection legislation and could thus be used by anyone.

Cover image: www.ingimage.com

This book is a translation from the original published under ISBN 978-620-6-70098-2.

Publisher:
Sciencia Scripts
is a trademark of
Dodo Books Indian Ocean Ltd. and OmniScriptum S.R.L publishing group

120 High Road, East Finchley, London, N2 9ED, United Kingdom
Str. Armeneasca 28/1, office 1, Chisinau MD-2012, Republic of Moldova, Europe
Printed at: see last page
ISBN: 978-620-7-54700-5

DEDICACES

I dedicate this work :

-To my father Noumou Doumbia

You, Dad, with whom I began this journey with a heart full of enthusiasm, and without whom I would never have had the courage and strength I needed. You have become the invisible hand that pushes me forward. After all these years, here today is the fruit of your labours, this work belongs to you.

May God bless you, Dad, and keep you healthy and alive for as long as possible by our side.

-To my mother Korotoumou Kanté

Thank you for the precious gift of life. You are the definition of a fighting woman in my eyes and my role model. The education you gave us was exemplary, you taught us to be self-reliant, rather than giving us fish, you taught us how to catch them.

Be honored on this day, Mom, because this modest work is but a small token of my deep gratitude and love.

May God keep you healthy and close to us for many years to come.

-To my grandmother

The late Nayouma Konaté thank you for your constant blessings. May Allah grant you paradise.

-To my brothers and sisters

Oumar, Sali, Moussa dit N'fa, Natenin, Mansa, the twins (Fatoumata and Adiaratou) and Mamadou. Dear brothers and sisters, this work is yours. Thank you for your kind and trusting affection. May Allah grant you long life and good health.

ACKNOWLEDGEMENTS

-A-ALLAH

God the Almighty, the Clement and the Merciful for having lent me long life, for having facilitated and granted the necessary means to complete this work. Ya Allah continues to guide my steps.

-To our prophet Mohamed

Peace and salvation upon him, upon all his family and companions, and upon all those who follow him until the Last Judgment.

-To the Konaté family at G

Issa Konaté, Moussa Konaté, the late Mariam Konaté, Oumou, Mayini ,Hawa, and especially Siratiki Konaté ,A man of sharing, love and kindness. Thank you for opening the doors of your home to me, where I was warmly welcomed and immediately felt like part of a family. Your generosity and advice enabled me to concentrate solely on what was essential, i.e. studying. Bless you for your generosity and good heart. May God watch over you and your whole family.

My aunts and uncles

Kadidiatou Kanté, Docteur Mamadou Kanté, Oumou Kanté, Nawasa Kanté, Marama Kanté, Fatoumata Kanté etc.

You have always been a support throughout my studies, your advice and prayers have been a great help to me, may God keep you.

To my friends and comrades of the twelfth numerus clausus class Sékou djiré, Kassim Niambéle, Oumar Samake, Oumar N'fal Dembélé, Youba Koita , yakana Cissé, Mamadou Doucoure, Mohamed yiriba Diarra , Docteur Ismaiel Konaté , Docteur Mahamadou Kané and the late Adama Diakité. May this work express my deepest gratitude for the help they have never failed to give me, and assure them of my friendly remembrance.

The CHME-Le Luxembourg ophthalmology and nephrology team

- **To Dr Diallo Oumar, Head of the Ophthalmology Department**

Thank you for welcoming me into your department to carry out this work. Your availability, your generosity, your scientific rigor and your love for a job well done make you an exemplary teacher.

Thank you so much for your guidance and advice, and thank you for your financial support. May Allah reward you for everything.

- **To Dr Djiguiba Karamoko, Head of the Nephrology Department**

Thank you for welcoming me into your department to carry out this work. You are a cultured, tolerant and understanding man. You have contributed a lot to my training, thank you for your advice on life in general, thank you for your support and your blessings.

- **Dr Fatoumata Traore**

Thank you for your generosity, assistance and involvement in the realization of this work.

Please find here, dear doctor, the expression of my deep gratitude and recognition.

My masters

- **Dr Berthé Kadidiatou**

Your good humor and contagious joie de vivre make our training easier and make you an exemplary teacher. Thank you for your availability and all the teachings you have given us. May God give you what your heart desires.

- **Dr Yacouba Coulibaly**

An exceptional elder, friend and advisor. Your support and trust have been a great help to me. May Allah reward you for everything.

- **Dr Haidara Mahalmoudou**

Your intellectual qualities, your generosity and your open-mindedness make you a person appreciated by all.

- **Dr Raphael Togo**

Thank you for your availability and, above all, your advice, which has helped to fuel my thinking. Your human qualities and commitment to patients make you an exemplary teacher.

Dr Traore Adama, Dr Tairou Traore , Docteur Doumbia Sory Ibrahim Mamadou Kané, Moussa Balla Dembélé ,Doukas Nassogo, Falaye Dembele Mamadou Touré, Mohamed Dembélé, Rokia Sylla, Mariam Bagayoko, Aboucar Diallo, Mariam Diallo etc.

To all those I forgot to mention, I may have forgotten on paper, but my heart hasn't forgotten a thing.

ABBREVIATIONS

NSAID: Non-steroidal anti-inflammatory drug

ALFEDIAM: French-language association for diabetes and metabolic diseases

AVL/SC: Uncorrected distance visual acuity

AVL/AC: Corrected distance visual acuity

AVP: Presence visual acuity

BAV: Baisse d'Acuité Visuelle CE: Corps Etrange

CHME: Centre Hospitalier Mère et Enfants (Mother and Child Hospital)

CRP: Protéine C réactive (C-reactive protein)

DFG: Débit de Filtration Glomérulaire (Glomerular filtration rate)

DPS: Débit pompes sanguins (Blood pump flow)

E.R.E.: extra-renal purification

FAV: arteriovenous fistula

F.O: Eye background

GB :Globules Blanc

GNRP: Rapidly progressive glomerulonephritis

Hb: Hemoglobin

HD: Hemodialysis

HTA: Hypertension HTO: Hypertonia Intra Ocular

HVB: Hepatitis B virus

HVC: Hepatitis C virus

HIV: Human Immunodeficiency Virus

IgG: Immunoglobin type G

IL2: Interleukin 2

IOTA: Institut d'Ophtalmologie Tropicale d'Afrique (Tropical Ophthalmology

Institute of Africa) IR: Insufficient renal function

AKI : Acute renal failure

CKD : Chronic renal failure

KT/F : Femoral venous catheter

KT/V: Venous catheter

SLE: Systemic lupus erythematosus

 CSF: Cerebrospinal fluid

OAP: Acute pulmonary oedema

OM: Macular edema

WHO: World Health Organization

PCP: pulmonary central pressure

IOP: Intraocular pressure

PPID: Weight gain between dialysis

Plq: Platelets

POμ:Phosphoremia

PTH: Parathormone

PVC: Central venous pressure

RD: Diabetic retinopathy

RDNP: Non-proliferative diabetic retinopathy

RH: Hypertensive retinopathy

S.A: Anterior segment

S.P: Posterior segment

TNF: Tumor necrosis factor

TPHA/VDRL: Treponema pallidum Haemagglutination Assay / Venereal

Disease Research Laboratory (syphilis screening test)

VA: arterial route

VIT: vitamin D

Table of contents

DEDICACES 1

ACKNOWLEDGEMENTS 2

ABBREVIATIONS 5

I-Introduction 8

II- Objectives : 10

III-   General : 11

IV-   METHODOLOGY 35

V-   Results 1-Frequency 49

VI-   COMMENTS AND DISCUSSION 60

VII-   Conclusion 63

VIII-   RECOMMENDATIONS 64

IX-   REFERENCES 65

X-   Appendices : 69

I-Introduction

Ocular complications in chronic hemodialysis patients are the indirect consequences of extra-renal purification (corneoconjunctival thesaurosis and retinopathy; retinal serous detachment; cataract) [6].

Chronic renal failure (CRF) corresponds to a decline over time in the number of functional nephrons, and usually becomes clinically evident only when creatinine clearance falls below 30ml/min [1]. The kidney plays a vital role in eliminating toxins, maintaining hydroelectrolyte homeostasis and acid-base balance. It also produces erythropoietin, the active vitamin D, and renin. [2].

Worldwide, around 1.3 million people die each year from kidney failure, with a further 1.4 million deaths due to cardiovascular disease attributed to impaired renal function; the prevalence of CKD is increasing at an alarming rate. Deaths due to CKD rose by 41.5% between 1990 and 2020, from the 17^e to the 10^e cause of death [3]. CKD is implicated in 4 to 22% of deaths in tropical Africa [4].

However, hemodialysis or extra-renal excretion (E.R.E.) is a technique for supplementing renal function. This method replaces deficient renal function [2].

In Morocco, studies carried out on ocular manifestations in haemodialysis patients in Casablanca in 2020 reported a frequency of 53% conjunctival hyperhaemia in the anterior segment (S.A) and retinopathy (23.07% hypertensive and 11.5% diabetic) in the posterior segment (S.P) [7]. Another study carried out in RABAT in 2021 found 40% cataracts in the S.A and 45% hypertensive retinopathy in the S.P [2].

In Cameroon in 2018, a frequency of 11.4% of severe lacrimal hyposecretion was reported in chronic hemodialysis patients [8].

In Mali, in 2019 at CHU-IOTA out of 32 haemodialysis patients, 34.37% of cataracts were reported on S.A involvement, 50% of hypertensive retinopathy (H.R.) on S.P involvement [9].

Improved dialysis techniques are prolonging the survival of dialysis patients, leading to the emergence of multiple cardiovascular and metabolic pathologies, with imbalances in phosphocalcic metabolism and anaemia causing ophthalmological damage tthe various segments of the eye [2].

Indeed, in order to have recent data on the follow-up of haemodialysis patients, it was necessary to study ocular complications in chronic haemodialysis patients at the Centre Hospitalier Universitaire Mère Enfant le Luxembourg, hence the interest of this thesis, which has the following objectives:

II- Objectives :

General objective

Study of ocular complications in hemodialysis patients at CHME Le Luxembourg.

Specific objectives

➢ To determine the socio-demographic characteristics of patients with ocular complications in haemodialysis patients at the CHME le Luxembourg.

➢ To describe the epidemiological and clinical aspects of ocular complications in hemodialysis patients at CHME Le Luxembourg.

➢ Describe the causal relationship between ocular complications and renal failure

III- General information :

A-Remind physiology and anatomy of the kidney and eye 1-Kidneys

The kidney is a thoracoabdominal organ, located behind the abdominal wall; the right kidney is slightly lower than the left to accommodate the location of the liver [10]. The two kidneys are bean-shaped, measuring approximately 12 centimetres in height, 6 centimetres in width and 3 centimetres in thickness. They are the starting point of the urinary system. These organs are in constant operation: the nephrons, tiny structures within the Malpighian pyramids, filter liters of blood every day. The kidneys reabsorb vital substances, remove undesirable elements and return the filtered blood to the body. And as if they weren't already busy enough, the kidneys also produce the urine that eliminates all waste products!

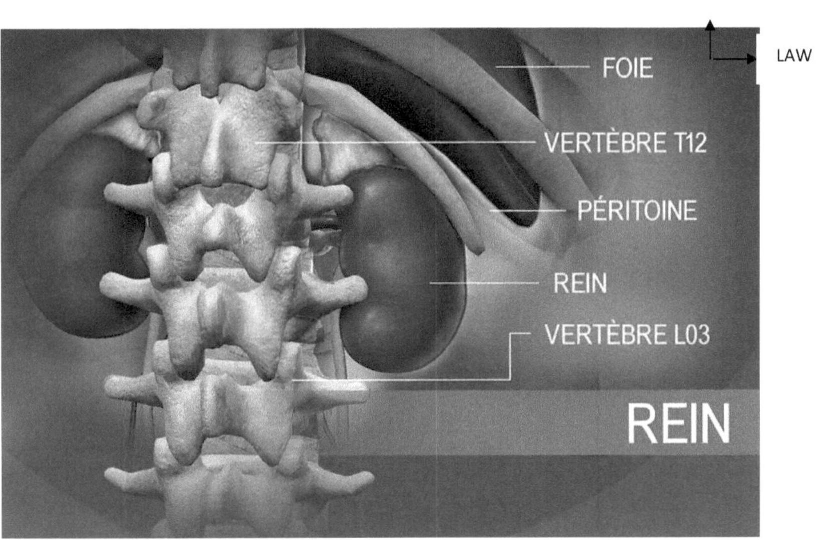

Figure 1: Location of right and left kidneys [11].

- Blood circulation inside and outside the kidneys

The arteries branch off into tiny capillaries that interact with the urinary structures in the kidneys: the nephrons. This is where the blood is filtered. Waste products are removed from the blood, and vital substances are reabsorbed and returned to the bloodstream. The filtered blood is rerouted via the renal veins. All the blood in the body passes through the kidneys hundreds of times a day; this corresponds to around 190 liters of filtered blood every 24 hours.

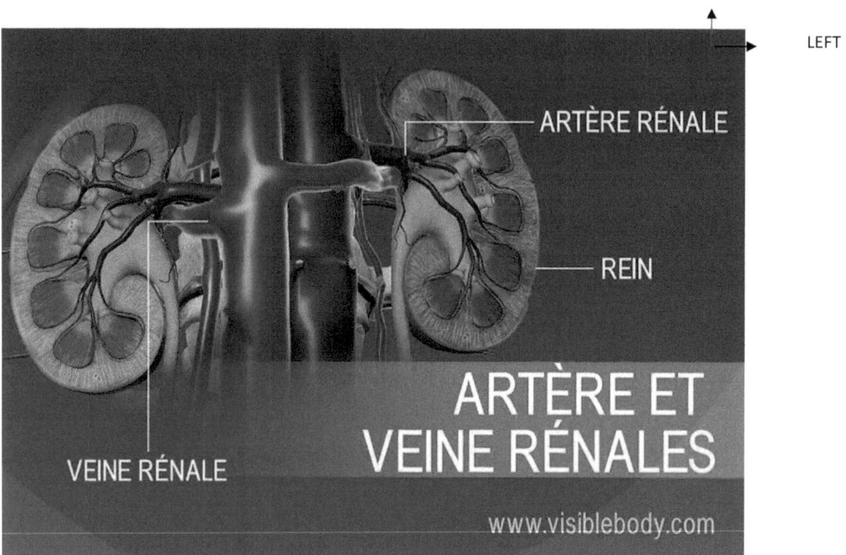

Figure 2: sagittal section of the right and left kidney showing blood flow and outside [11].

-The three main sections of the kidneys

Each kidney consists of an outer renal cortex, an inner renal medulla and a renal pelvis. Blood is filtered in the renal cortex. The renal medullary contains the Malpighian pyramids, where urine is formed.

Urine passes from the Malpighian pyramids to the renal pelvis. This funnel-shaped structure occupies the central cavity of each kidney, then narrows as it stretches to join the ureter. Urine flows from the renal pelvis into the ureter.

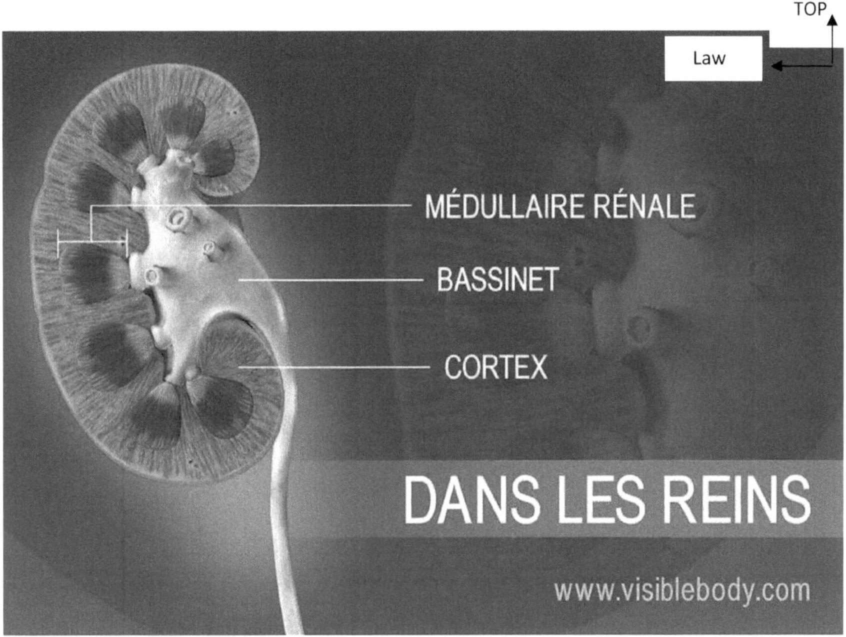

Figure 3: sagittal section of the right kidney showing the internal configuration [11].

- **Nephrons**: the fundamental functional units of blood filtration and urine production. Each kidney contains over a million tiny structures called nephrons. They are located partly in the cortex and partly inside the Malpighian pyramids, where their tubules make up most of the pyramid mass.

Nephrons perform the primary function of the kidneys: they regulate the concentration of water and other substances in the body. They filter blood, reabsorb what the body needs, and excrete the rest in the form of urine.

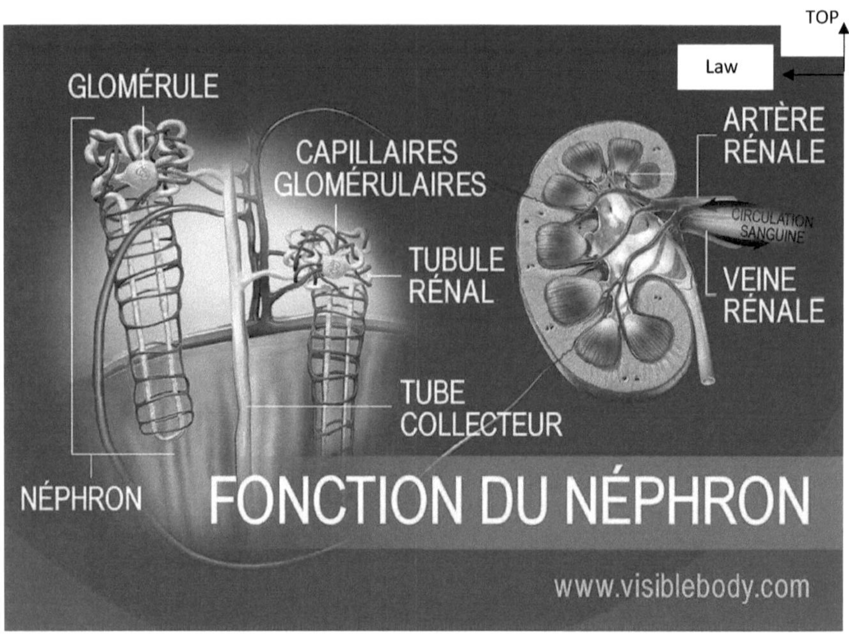

Figure 4: sagittal section of the right kidney showing the structure of the nephron [11].

2- THE EYE

The eyeball is a spherical organ located in the orbit and responsible for visual function. Its average length is 24 mm, its weight 7 g and its volume 6.5 cm. It is made up of three envelopes: the sclera (outer envelope), the uvea (intermediate envelope) and the retina (inner envelope).

It contains three transparent media: the aqueous humor, the crystalline lens and the vitreous body. It is divided into two segments:

The anterior segment is the space between the cornea and the posterior surface of the lens. From front to back, we find the cornea, the anterior chamber with the aqueous humor, the iris and the lens.

The posterior segment is the space behind the lens. From front to back, we distinguish the vitreous cavity with the vitreous humor, the retina, the choroid and the sclera.

Eye movements are p e r f o r m e d by the oculomotor muscles. The annexes are the eyelids and lacrimal ducts.

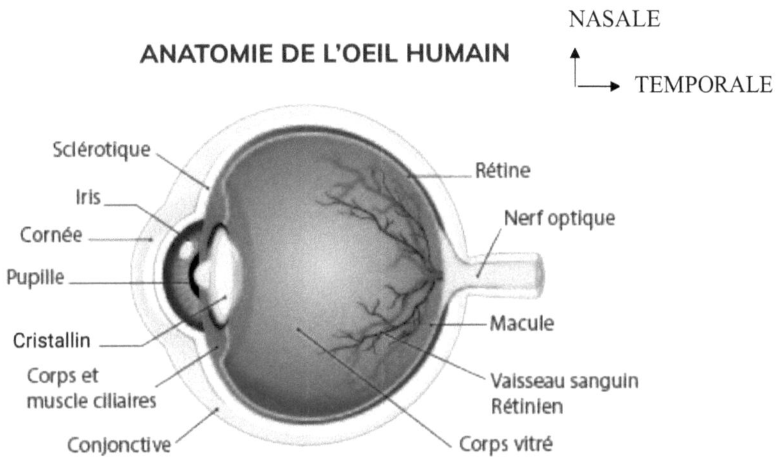

Figure 5: sagittal section of the eyeball [12].

The cornea :

The cornea is the transparent front part of the eyeball. It is embedded in an opening in the sclera. It is the eye's primary refractive element accounting for ⅔ of the ocular dioptre, with the crystalline lens making up the remaining 1/3. It measures around 530 microns in thickness.

It consists of five layers:

• The corneal surface epithelium: in contact with the tear film, it is made up of three cell layers: the basal layer, the intermediate layer and the superficial layer.

• Bowman's membrane: acellular layer between the corneal epithelium and stroma.

• The stroma accounts for 90% of corneal thickness. It is made up of a fundamental substance, collagen fibers, keratocytes and fibrocytes.

- Descemet's membrane: transparent, amorphous, elastic basal membrane. It lies between the stroma and the corneal endothelium.

- The endothelium: a monolayer of aregenerative cells in contact with the aqueous humor. Its main function is to maintain a constant state of hydration in the corneal stroma, compatible with the cornea's physiological role of transmitting light.

The main characteristic of the cornea is its lack of vascularization. It draws its nourishment from the limbus, the tear film and the aqueous humor.

Iris:

The iris is the most anterior part of the uvea, following on from the ciliary body. It is a pigmented, circular, contractile membrane, bulging forward and perforated at its center by an orifice: the pupil.

The iris has two edges:

- An external peripheral one that inserts onto the ciliary body

- The inner one delimits the pupil

Pupil contraction and dilation are controlled by two antagonistic muscles:

- The pupillary sphincter muscle

- The pupillary dilator muscle

The physiological pupillary reflex uses these muscles to adapt vision to ambient light.

We speak of myosis when the pupil is contracted and mydriasis when the pupil is dilated.

Aniridia is the absence of the iris.

Heterochromia is a difference in color between the two eyes or between parts of the same eye.

The iris separates the anterior chamber from the posterior chamber.

Iridocorneal angle:

The iridocorneal angle is delimited by the anterior surface of the iris and the posterior surface of the cornea. It contains several elements whose main function is the excretion of aqueous humor:

- Schwable ring: condensation of the Descemet membrane.
- The trabeculum: a meshwork of collagen fibers responsible for aqueous humor filtration. Dysfunction of the trabeculum leads to an increase in intraocular pressure through reduced filtration of aqueous humor.
- Schlemm's canal: excretory pathway for aqueous humor.

The ciliary body

The ciliary body is the intermediate segment of the circular uvea, located behind the iris, and consists of two structures:

- The ciliary muscle, which plays a role in accommodation and corresponds to the insertion zone of the iris root and zonule.
- The ciliary processes are richly vascularized and composed of ciliary epithelium. They play a major role in the secretion of aqueous humor.

The lens :

The crystalline lens is a biconvex lens, the eye's second refractive element after the cornea. It accounts for a third of the ocular dioptre, and has a normal refractive power of 13 diopters. The crystalline lens lies behind the iris and is attached to the eye's envelope by the zonules at the ciliary bodies. It is composed of a nucleus, a cortex and an anterior and posterior capsule. It is transparent, without vascularization or innervation. With age, the various structures of the lens can become opaque, leading to cataracts. The crystalline lens is able to contract thanks to the zonules under the effect of the ciliary muscle, enabling it to play its role in accommodation. The loss of this accommodative function is progressive over time and is responsible for presbyopia.

Sclera:

The sclera, the outermost layer of the eyeball, corresponds to the resistant opaque white membrane occupying ⅘ of the globe's surface. Its structure is tendinous and acellular, and its thickness varies from 1 to 2 mm.

Its main role is to maintain the shape, tone and integrity of the globe. The optic nerve runs through the back of the eye, while vessels and nerves run along the sides. The anterior part is covered by the conjunctiva. The oculomotor muscles are inserted here.

The conjunctive :

The conjunctiva is the transparent mucous membrane lining the anterior surface of the sclera (bulbar conjunctiva) and the inner surface of the eyelids (tarsal conjunctiva), with the bulbar and tarsal parts mirroring each other at the conjunctival culs de sac.

Histologically, the epithelium contains caliciform cells responsible for mucus secretion.

The retina

The retina, the sensitive organ of vision, extends and covers the entire inner surface of the choroid down to the Ora errata. Its main function is phototransduction. To the front, the retina is in contact with the vitreous humor, and to the rear with the choroid.

There are three special zones:

- The macula: central area of the retina
- The fovea: central depression of the macula characterized by a high density of cones, where visual acuity is at its best
- Lapapilleoptique : area o f   emergence of   a photoreceptor-free infopticulus.   photoreceptors .

The retina is made up of two tissues:

- The neurosensory layer: made up of cones and rods: photoreceptors that capture light signals and transform them into electrochemical signals.
- The pigment epithelium, which has four main roles: as a screen, in

exchanges, in vitamin A metabolism, and in phagocytosis of photoreceptor outer articles.

From a histological point of view, 10 layers can be distinguished, from exterior to interior:

- Pigment epithelium
- The photoreceptor layer includes cones, which are responsible focentral and color vision, and rods, which are responsible for peripheral and night vision.
- The outer limiting membrane
- The outer nuclear layer
- The outer plexiform layer
- The inner nuclear layer
- The inner plexiform layer
- The ganglion cell layer
- The optical fiber layer
- The internal limiting membrane

The choroid

The choroid is the nourishing membrane of the eye. It forms a vascular sponge between the retina and the sclera, and is made up of numerous pigmented cells and vascular-nervous elements. It extends from the optic disc to the ciliary bodies. The long and short posterior ciliary arteries, the verticose veins and the ciliary nerves run through it.

Le vitré

With a gel-like structure in the center and fibrous at the periphery, the vitreous occupies ⅘ of the ocular volume, or 4ml. It acts as a buffer for the retina and as a site for exchanges with the various neighboring structures. It is surrounded by a thin membrane called the hyaloid, lining the inner face of the retina Any traction of the vitreous fibers from the base of the vitreous can tear the retina and detach it.

The eyelids

The eyelids cover the anterior part of the eyeball, and are responsible for protecting the eyeball, lacrimal drainage and mimic expression. They are cutaneous, muscular and fibrous, and are richly vascularized and innervated.

Anatomically, from outside to inside, we find :

- A layer of skin on the outside
- A fibro-elastic framework
- A muscular plan
- A tarsal conjunctiva covering the inner surface

The eyelids are vascularized by the internal and external carotid arteries.

The facial nerve (nerve VII), the oculomotor nerve (nerve III), the trigeminal nerve (nerve V) and the sympathetic nerve from the upper cervical ganglion contribute to motor and sensory innervation of the eyelids.

There are two rows of eyelashes on their free edge and around thirty Meibomius glands on each eyelid.

The oculomotor muscles

The oculomotor muscular system comprises 6 muscles:

4 straight muscles :

Superior rectus innervated by nerve III Inferior rectus innervated by nerve III Medial rectus innervated by nerve III

The lateral rectus muscle innervated by nerve VI 2 oblique muscles :

The superior oblique muscle innervated by nerve IV The inferior oblique muscle innervated by nerve III **The lacrimal system**

Tears are secreted by the lacrimal glands and form the lacrimal lake in the lower conjunctival cul-de-sac.

They pass through :

- Upper and lower tear points
- Upper and lower canaliculi

- The common canaliculus
- The lacrimal sac
- The nasolacrimal canaliculus
- The Hanser valve
- To drain into the nasal cavity

Tearing is a characteristic sign of lacrimal duct obstruction.

Obstruction of the lacrimal duct leads to lacrimation, which can be complicated by an infection of the lacrimal sac known as acute dacryocystitis [12].

B- the oculo-renal correlation in the manifestations and mechanisms of many diseases :

The development of interdisciplinary cooperation in clinical, biochemical and genetic fields has led to the discovery of an oculo-renal correlation in the manifestations and mechanisms of numerous diseases [13].

There are many morbid associations between the eye and the kidney, despite their different embryonic origins: mesoderm for the kidney, ectoderm for the eye.

Their organogenesis runs parallel in time, with an initial critical period between the fourth and sixth weeks of development. Abnormalities in embryogenesis can affect both organs. The proximity of certain genes also explains why they can be affected together by chromosomal abnormalities, such as the association between Wilms' tumor and aniridia.

The structural kinship between certain parts of the kidney and the eye also accounts for many eye-kidney pathological correlations: Bruch's basement membrane and that of renal glomeruli affected by IgG deposits in Good Pasture syndrome and in certain membrano-proliferative glomerulonephritis, type IV collagen abnormalities in glomerular nephropathy and lens damage in Alport syndrome, identity of the extracellular matrix of the cornea and mesangium, arachidonic acid metabolites regulate water flow in the cornea and Henle's loop, crystalline fiber membrane channels for water transport are identical to those of tubular cells, cross-reactivity with retinal S antigen of regulatory proteins of membrane receptors coupled to glomerular and tubular cell proteins.

Certain pathogenic processes affect the eye and kidney in the same way: vasculitis in periarthritis nodosa , lymphoplasmacytic infiltrate in Gougerot-Sjogren's syndrome , deposits (amyloidosis , cystinosis ...) .

Finally, the eye suffers from kidney dysfunction: chronic renal failure, nephropathy with hypertension. Certain pathologies, such as hypertension, gout, sickle cell anemia and Waldenstrom's disease, affect the eye and kidney simultaneously.

The ophthalmological manifestations observed during CKD are mainly described in dialysis patients, and it is sometimes difficult to distinguish between complications that are dialysis-related and those that are CKD-related.

This is why their description is grouped together. They are part of a group of clinical disorders whose expression and intensity vary from patient to patient. They are rarely highlighted in general descriptions of CKD, despite the frequency of some of them. High blood pressure and disturbances in phosphocalcium metabolism are the main factors.

Hypertension is virtually constant in the terminal stage. It was already present if the initial nephropathy was glomerular. It aggravates CKD through the vascular and arteriolar lesions it induces. Disturbances in phosphocalcium metabolism occur early, even if their clinically obvious consequences are delayed. Hyperphosphatemia, hypocalcemia, vitamin D deficiency and hyperparathyroidism are the main features. When the solubility limits of the calcium-phosphorus product are exceeded, ubiquitous metastatic calcifications occur, leading to clinical manifestations when they are located in the conjunctiva (conjunctival hyperemia resulting in the red eye of chronic renal failure).

Since 1960, periodic hemodialysis has enabled many patients with end-stage CKD to enjoy prolonged survival. However, renal function replacement is imperfect, as evidenced by the following symptoms

- **Refractive disorders :**

Very common 30% are largely responsible for VAD in hemodialysis patients.

-**Corneo-conjunctival damage:**

Calcium deposits are the main ocular complication of CKD, affecting 50% of patients. These phosphocalcic disorders appear to be compounded by a dialysis-dependent factor, since the percentage of patients affected increases with the total number of dialysis sessions. Some authors distinguish dystrophic calcifications of the anterior segment from those known as <<metastatic >>.

Although most often asymptomatic, these calcium deposits can irritate the corneo-conjunctival epithelium, causing redness of the eye.

Other corneal changes caused by calcium overload, such as limbal Vogt degeneration and strip keratitis, are frequently observed in chronic renal failure.

Subconjunctival hemorrhage is sometimes the result of a uremic or heparin-induced hemorrhagic diathesis.

-**Cataracts :**

This is an uncommon complication of CKD: from small crystalline opacities to total cataracts, the evolution depends on phosphocalcic disturbances, age, duration of hemodialysis, and long-term corticosteroid therapy for pre-existing nephropathy. The role of oxidative stress in renal failure has been suggested.

- **Ocular hypertonia:**

Coupled with increased CSF pressure, it can mar the course of hemodialysis, causing headaches and nausea. It is linked to a change in the molar bone gradient between plasma on the one hand, and aqueous humor and CSF on the other, as a result of delayed elimination of one of these two fluid compartments. These pressure variations can be reduced by more frequent high-flow dialysis sessions. The use of dextrose and renal ultrafiltration can help lower IOP and intracranial pressure. An acute episode of glaucoma should be treated with myotic eye drops, beta-blockers and carbonic anhydrase inhibitors.

-Posterior segment disorders :

FO pallor due to anemia and retinal edema in hypertensive retinopathy are the most frequent manifestations of posterior segment damage in these patients.

Hypertensive retinopathy may improve on hemodialysis. Most chorio-retinal and papillary alterations are not a specific clinical entity and result from hypertension, arteriosclerosis, anemia or molar bone disturbances during dialysis sessions: retinal or papillary ischemia, papilledema, cystoid macular edema, retinal hemorrhages or exudative retinal detachment.

Chronic arterial hypotension and atheroma, common in dialysis patients, can lead to thrombosis of the central retinal artery. Retinopathy similar to Purtscher's retinopathy is a recognized cause of sudden blindness in hemodialysis patients. The hypothesized mechanism is leukoembolization of retinal arterioles following complement activation.

This type of retinopathy can be observed in CKD outside the context of hemodialysis. Bullous retinal detachments associated with serous detachments have been described in hemodialysis patients[1,5,7,14,15].

Table I: Classification of hypertensive retinopathy according to KirKendall [1].

Classification de Kirkendall		
	Rétinopathie hypertensive	**Artériosclérose**
I	Rétrécissement artériel	Signe du croisement
II	Stade I + : - hémorragies rétiniennes - nodules cotonneux - "exsudats secs"	Signe du croisement + rétrécissement artériel en regard
III	Stade II + œdème papillaire	Stade II + : - engainements vasculaires - occlusion de branche veineuse

Table II: ALFEDIAM classification of diabetic retinopathy [1].

Classification de la rétinopathie diabétique selon l'ALFEDIAM	
Pas de rétinopathie	
RD non proliférante	Minime
	Modérée
	Sévère ou pré proliférante
RD proliférante	Minime
	Modérée
	Sévère
	Compliquée
Maculopathie œdémateuse	Exsudats entourant l'OM
	OM diffus de la région centrale
Maculopathie ischémique	

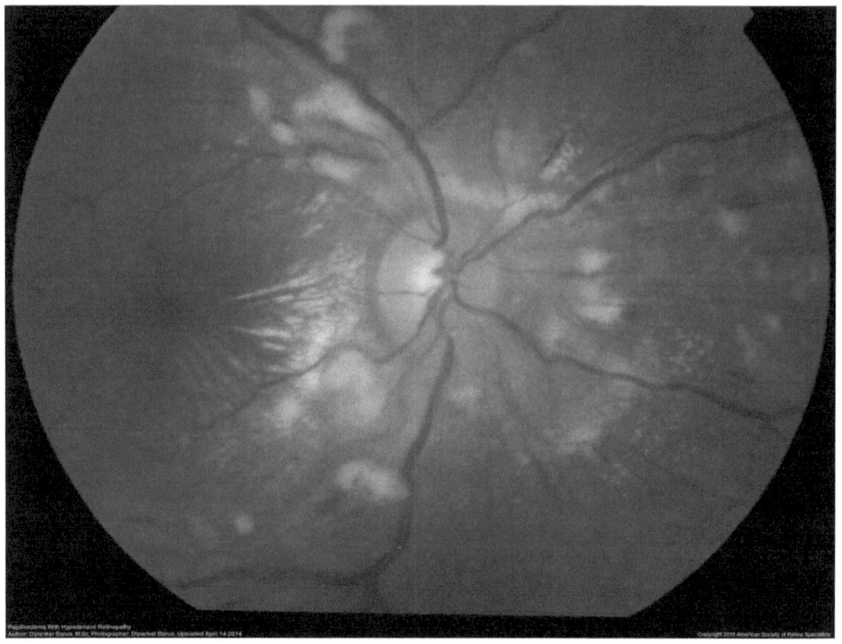

Figure 6: Severe hypertensive retinopathy of a right eye [16].

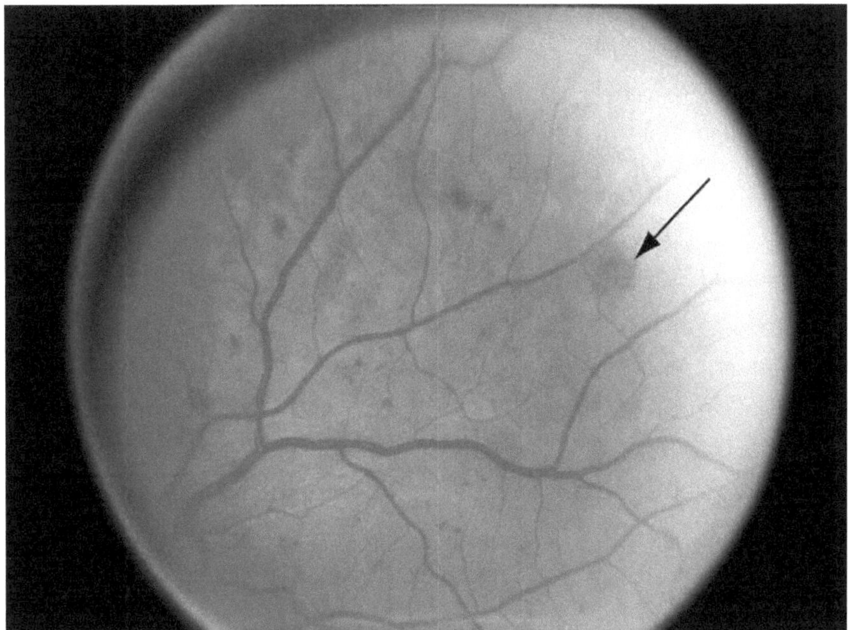

Figure 7: Retinophotograph showing diffuse intraretinal haemorrhages (arrow) and micro-aneurysms in non-proliferative diabetic retinopathy (NPDR) [17].

-Manifestations - neuro-ophthalmological :

Dialysis-enhanced ophthalmology of unknown but probably toxic mechanism may be observed in isolation or associated with Wernicke's encephalopathy in chronic dialysis patients (thiamine deficiency of multiple causes). Ischemic optic neuropathies have also been described.

- Ocular complications in chronic renal failure are :

- Refractive disorders.
- Retinopathies (hypertensive, diabetic, mixed).
- Cataracts.
- Corneo-conjunctival deposits.
- Ocular hypertonia.
- Optic neuropathies.

-       Arterial and venous vascular thrombosis.

-       And dry syndrome. [1,5,714,15]

C- HEMODIALYSIS

1- Definition

This is an exchange of solutes and water between the patient's blood and a dialysis solution with a composition similar to that of normal extracellular fluid, through a semi-permeable membrane.

2-   Goal

Its purpose is to eliminate waste products and maintain the body's hydroelectrolytic balance.

3-   Hemodialysis theory:

The transfer of solutes and water involves two fundamental mechanisms

These are diffusion or conduction and convection or ultrafiltration, to which transfer is added.

3-1- Diffusion or conduction :

Transfer by diffusion or conduction is the passive transport of solutes from the blood to the dialysate through the dialysis membrane, without the passage of solvent. It depends on 3 factors: the diffusion coefficient of the solute in the blood, the dialysis membrane and the dialysate.

3-2- Convection or ultrafiltration :

This is the simultaneous transfer of the solvent and a fraction of the solutes it contains under the effect of a difference in hydrostatic pressure. It can take place either from the blood compartment to the dialysate, or from the dialysate to the blood.

It also depends on 3 factors: the membrane sieving coefficient, the average plasma solute concentration and the solvent filtration rate.

3-3- Transfer :

Convective transfer results in the simultaneous subtraction of solutes and solvent (water, sodium), whereas diffusion transfer only allows the passage of solutes (waste substance). Ultrafiltration is the only mechanism by which water and sodium accumulated between two dialysis sessions are removed from the body.

3-4- Osmosis :

This is the transfer of solvent under the effect of an osmotic pressure difference. As the plasma passes through the dialyzer, its protein concentration rises due to the loss of water through filtration, thus increasing the osmotic pressure of the plasma at the dialyzer outlet.

This results in the osmotic transfer of water and solutes from the intracellular sector to the interstitial sector and plasma, restoring circulating blood volume.

3-5- Adsorption :

Proteins such as albumin, fibrin, beta 2 micro globulin, active complement fragments and cytokines such as IL2 and TNF can, to a certain extent, be adsorbed onto the dialysis membrane. The same applies to strongly protein-bound substances such as hemocysteine.

This mechanism contributes, in part, to their extraction from the blood. This is an exclusive property of hydrophobic membranes.

3-6- The concentration gradient :

It is the difference in concentration of a given substance in two liquid compartments separated by a semi-permeable membrane. The dialyzer comprises two compartments, one bloody and the other liquid, the dialysis bath. The creation of a difference in concentration of the substances to be eliminated in these 2 compartments is therefore necessary for the different physical properties, diffusion and osmosis, to take place.

The creation of a concentration gradient is the basis of dialysis. Blood contains the waste products of nitrogen metabolism (urea, creatinine, uric acid) as well as water and electrolytes. The dialysis bath contains no waste products. The movement of urea and other waste products is always from the blood into the dialysis bath. The purified blood returns to the patient, where it mixes with the total blood volume. It will also be loaded with degradation products from the body's other fluid compartments. Thus, when it passes through the dialyzer, the rate of eliminated substance is roughly equal to that of the first pass. By successive passages through the artificial kidney, a significant quantity of degradation products is extracted from the blood, bringing its composition closer to normal.

3-7-Dialysis membrane :

Dialysis membranes are designed to reproduce as closely as possible the permeability characteristics of the glomerular basement membrane. Cellulose membranes, either unsubstituted like cuprophan or substituted like homophone or cellulose di- and triacetate, are hydrophilic, whereas synthetic polymeric membranes are hydrophobic. Newer membranes made from copolymers are both hydrophobic and hydrophilic, enhancing both their diffusion performance and their absorption capacity.

4-   Basic dialysis techniques :

The artificial kidney is a set of compact components comprising :

- A blood circuit.
- A dialysis bath circuit.
- A dialysis membrane or dialyzer.
- A dialysis machine.

5 -Indications for hemodialysis management in CKD: In CKD, the criterion for hemodialysis management is the creatinine clearance value. When this falls below 10 ml/min, treatment may be justified if the symptoms o f CKD become difficult to control with conservative treatment.

Below 5 ml/min, even in the absence of any symptoms, there is a definite need for dialysis, to avoid the rapid onset of serious problems associated with severe chronic uraemia (pericarditis, pulmonary oedema, weight loss, hyperkalaemia, etc.). When these problems arise, dialysis treatment is of course imperative.

In exceptional cases, management may be carried out before the CKD reaches a creatinine clearance value of 10 ml/min, for example when decompensated cardiac disease, which makes any excess of sodium and water intolerable, is added to the IR.

Similarly, in diabetics, it is recommended that patients be treated between 10 and 20ml/min creatinine clearance.

When the decision is made to use hemodialysis for CKD, it will almost always be definitive and therefore chronic.

Functional recovery can nevertheless sometimes be observed, for example when ultrafiltration enables cardiac reward and thus an improvement in a possible pre-renal component of CKD.

6-   Indications for hemodialysis management of ARF Hemodialysis should generally be considered within 48 to 72 hours of the acute event

Two criteria are then taken into account:

- Hydro-sodium overload assessed on the basis of arterial pressures and, above all, central venous and, if possible, pulmonary capillary pressures (even in the absence of peripheral edema).

The decision is generally taken when CVP exceeds 20 cmH2O or when PCP exceeds 20 mm Hg. OAP is a formal indication.

However, these patients should not be managed too quickly on the basis of this criterion alone, as the resumption of spontaneous diuresis depends on a certain degree of overload.

When only this criterion is present, the decision is made to reduce expansion of the extracellular space and avoid pulmonary oedema, but care is taken to maintain a small overload after the session, in order to maintain a certain pressure, which will enable the kidneys to recover more or less rapidly.

In exceptional cases, the decision to dialyze may be taken, for the reason of hydrosaline overload, in the absence of any hypertension or venous disease.

This is the case when significant peripheral edema is present, following marked protein hypo.

Dialysis is then carried out under albumin infusion.

- Controlled **hyperkalemia**, above at least 6.5 mEq/l, if accompanied by electrocardiographic manifestations (bradycardia, giant T wave, AV block, etc.) is a formal indication for dialysis, in the context of ARF. Other criteria may also be taken into account, but are not, on their own, formal criteria. These are uraemia and acidosis, which in fact only become formal criteria well after the first two in the course of ARF. Nevertheless, in the presence of oligo-anuria, the decision to dialyze may be taken for uraemia exceeding 3.5 g/l or for a bicarbonate standard below 10 mmol

/l, even in the absence of other criteria.

In recent years, new prognostic criteria have come into play, particularly in intensive care units, when it comes to deciding on acute hemodialysis management. These criteria are based on the evaluation of certain survival scores (Glasgow scores, Apache scores, etc.).

AKI that lasts longer than 48 hours (after which acute dialysis is usually considered), since tubular necrosis almost always occurs, whether primary or secondary.

7- Complications of dialysis a- Acute complications :

- Hypotension.

- Muscle cramps.

- Anaphylactic reactions to the dialyzer (bio-incompatible cellulose membranes).

b- Chronic complications :

- **Cardiovascular complications** :

Hypertension, ischemic heart disease, pericarditis, left ventricular failure, endocarditis, valvulopathy.

- **Osteoarticular complications :**

Renal osteodystrophy, amyloidosis

- **Hepatobiliary complications :**

Hepatitis, ulcers and constipation.

- **Skin complications:**

Pruritus, dry skin, purpura, bilious dermatosis or pseudoporphyria cutanea tarda, cutaneous necrosis, hypertrichosis, acne.

- **Hematological complications :**

Anemia, hemolysis, polycythemia, hyperplaquettosis, iron overload, hemostasis disorders.

- **Neurological complications :**

Aluminic encephalopathy, imbalance syndrome, intracerebral hemorrhage, chronic dementia, sleep disorders, carpal tunnel syndrome, impatient legs syndrome, autonomic neuropathy, convulsions.

- **Infectious complications :**

They are the second most common cause of death in hemodialysis patients, accounting for up to 38% of all deaths. The most frequent are: septicemia, bronchopulmonary infections, ENT and dental infections, genitourinary infections, skin and soft tissue infections, osteoarticular infections and tuberculosis.

- **Ocular complications :**

Refractive disorders, cataracts, corneoconjunctival deposits, intraocular hypertonia (IOH), optic neuropathies, arterial and venous vascular thromboses, dry syndrome, retinopathies (hypertensive, diabetic, mixed) are the focus of our study [5,4,18,19,20] **D- Drugs and the eye**

Certain medications sometimes used in dialysis patients can cause eye problems:

Sulfonamides: keratoconjunctivitis associated with erythema, Stevens Johnson syndrome.

Quinine and quinidine: maculopathy. NSAIDs: toxic amblyopia, retinopathy.

Corticoids: cataracts, glaucoma (especially local applications), susceptibility to eye infections (herpes viruses, bacteria).

Ethambutol: BAV, central scotoma, dyschromatopsia. Isoniazid: retrobulbar neuropathy.

Morphine: extreme myosis (overdose) [5,7,15].

IV- METHODOLOGY

1- Study framework:

The study took place in the ophthalmology and hemodialysis departments of the Centre Hospitalier Mère- Enfant (CHME) Le Luxembourg.

1-2 Hospital presentation

The Centre Hospitalier Universitaire Mère-Enfant (CHME) "Le Luxembourg" was inaugurated on November 24, 1998 and began operations in May 1999.

The CHME obtained its operating license under decree no. 02-1845/MS- SG of August 27, 2002. It is owned by the Fondation Amadou Toumani Touré Pour l'Enfance (FATTPE). This Foundation, headed by Madame Touré Lobo Traoré, is recognized as a public utility by Decree N° 93-271 PRM of August 06, 1993. The CHUME is located to the west of Bamako, in the Hamdallaye district, and covers an area of 3,461 m^2 .

On February 02, 2015, the center signed a partnership agreement with the rectorate of the Université des Sciences des Techniques et des Technologies de Bamako (USTTB), making it a Centre Hospitalier Universitaire (CHU).

In 2018, an agreement signed with the French association La Chaîne de l'Espoir (CdE) enabled the opening of the André FESTOC Center (CAF) for the care of children with heart disease in Mali. In the same year, another agreement signed with the Principality of Monaco and partners enabled the construction and equipping of a cardiac catheterization unit.

Thanks to the public utility status granted to the Foundation, it has signed an agreement with the Ministry of Health to manage the center, specifying the commitments of each party.

The Fondation Amadou Toumani Touré Pour l'Enfance through the Centre Hospitalier Universitaire Mere-Enfant "Le Luxembourg" undertakes to :

- Facilitate access to quality curative, preventive and promotional care in accordance with national health policy guidelines in the Republic of Mali;

- Provide patients at the CHME with INN drugs at affordable prices;

The Ministry of Health is committed to :

- Provide, within its means, the support the Foundation needs to achieve its objectives;

- To make available to the CHME "Le Luxembourg", at the Foundation's request, personnel corresponding to its needs. This staff, remunerated by the Ministry of Health, will be governed by the regulations governing the operation of the CHME "Le Luxembourg";

- Promote collaboration between CHME staff and other social and health workers in the department, and contracts with all health-related institutions and organizations.

1-2.1 Status

It is a 3ème level private Hospital Center under hospital law, not-for-profit and recognized as being of public utility. It became a University Hospital Center (CHU) on February 02, 2015, with the signing of an agreement with the rectorate of the University of Science, Techniques and Technologies of Bamako (USTTB).

1-2.2 CHME's missions

The CHME is a 3ème referral hospital open to patients referred by the CSRéfs, but also by 3ème level structures for cases requiring specialized intervention. As such, it has four main missions:

- Diagnose and treat patients, especially women and children;

- Manage referrals and emergencies;

- Continuing education for healthcare professionals and students;

- Conduct health-related research.

To carry out its missions and achieve its objectives, the CHME has set up several departments and services:

- Clinical Department,
- Medico-Technical Department,
- The Administrative Department,
- Support services.

1-2.3 Service organization

The Centre Hospitalier Universitaire Mère-Enfant "Le Luxembourg" is organized into eleven (11) departments comprising thirty-one (31) services, twenty-one (21) units and an accounting agency.

The departments are as follows:

A. Administrative and Financial Department ;
B. Department of Pediatrics;
C. Department of Gynecology and Obstetrics;
D. Department of Internal Medicine;
E. Department of Surgery;
F. The Department of Anesthesia, Intensive Care and Emergencies ;
G. Cardiology Department;
H. Department of Cardiovascular and Thoracic Surgery
I. Department of Pharmacy and Laboratory ;
J. Department of Radiology and Medical Imaging;
K. Department of Public Health.

Each department is organized into services, and the services into units according to the configuration of specialties.

A. Administrative and Financial Department

It is made up of five (05) departments and six (06) units:

1.	Department - Human Resources (HR) ;

2.	Service - Billing ;

3.	Social Service;

4.	Service - Maintenance.

5.	Accounting department :

a.	Unit - Material accounting

b.	Unit - Cost accounting

c.	Unit - Supply ;

6.	Secretariat Pool ;

7.	Surveillance Générale (SG) ;

8.	Hygiene and sanitation.

**B.	The Accounting Agency**

It comprises two (02) units:

1.	Treasury

2.	General accounting

**C.	Department of Pediatrics**

It comprises two (02) departments:

1.	General Pediatrics Department

2.	Neonatology department.

**D.	Department of Gynecology and Obstetrics**

It comprises two (02) departments and one (01) unit:

1.	Gynecology Department,

2.	Obstetrics Department.

a. Vaccination unit

**E.	Department of Internal Medicine**

It is made up of three (03) departments and six (08) units, as follows:

1.   Internal Medicine Department**;**

a.   Gastroenterology ;

b.   Endocrinology-Diabetology ;

c.   Infectiology ;

d.   Rheumatology ;

e.   Dermatology ;

f.   Neurology;

g.   Pneumology ;

2.   Nephrology Department;

a.   Hemodialysis unit.

3.   Medical Oncology Department.

F.   Department of Surgery

It is made up of six (06) departments and two (02) units as follows:

1.   General Surgery Department;

2.   Ophthalmology Department;

3.   Neurosurgery Department;

4.   Ear, Nose and Throat (ENT) Department;

5.   Traumatology and Orthopedics Department;

6.   Urology Department;

a.   Pediatric Surgery Unit;

b.   Odonto-stomatology unit.

G.   Department of Anesthesia, Intensive Care and Emergencies

It comprises four (04) departments:

1.   Anesthesia Department;

2.   Intensive Care Unit;

3.   The Emergency Department ;

4.   The Operating Theatre Department.

H.   Cardiology Department

It comprises two (02) departments:

1.   Cardiology department;

2.   Cardiac catheterization department.

I.   Department of Cardiovascular and Thoracic Surgery

It comprises two (02) departments:

1.   Cardiac surgery department;

2.   The vascular and thoracic surgery department.

J.   Laboratory Department - Pharmacy

It comprises two (02) departments:

1.   Laboratory services ;

2.   Hospital Pharmacy Department.

K.   Department of Public Health:

                        1. Department - Hospital Information System (HIS)

a.   Unit - Communication, Information, Documentation ;

b.   Unit - Medical Informatics

L.   Department of Radiology and Medical Imaging.

It comprises two (02) departments:

1.   Radiology Department

2.   Medical Imaging Department

3.

1-2.4 CHME management

The CHME is under the direct supervision of the Fondation Amadou Toumani Touré Pour l'Enfance. To ensure it operates smoothly, the CHME has the following administrative and management bodies:

o   the board of directors ;
o   general management ;
o   management committee ;
o   Institutional Medical Committee (CME);
o   Works council (CTE) ;
o   Health and Safety Technical Committee (CTHS);
o   Intra-hospital Death Audit Committee (CADIH);
o   Committee on Nursing and Obstetrics (CNO);
o   the haemovigilance committee.

1-2.5 CHME's partners

a- Local partners :

For better care coordination, CHME "Le Luxembourg" has developed a local partnership with :

o   Bamako and Kati District University Hospitals;
o   Reference Health Centres in Communes III and IV;
o   Direction Centrale du Service de Santé des Armées (DCSSA);
o   Université des Sciences, des Techniques et des Technologies de Bamako (USTTB);
o   Institut National de Formation en Sciences de la Santé (INFSS);
o   private training schools in the health sciences;

o   Orange Mali;

o   Banque Nationale du Développement Agricole (BNDA);

o   Pari Mutuel Urbain (PMU) Mali.

b- Approved structures :

o   The Embassy of the United States of America in Mali;

o   US-AID;

o   SANLAM Insurance;

o   la Mutualité Malienne ;

o   CANAM ;

o   ANAM;

o   Lycée Sportif de Kabala ;

o   Allianz Assurance ;

o   Atlantic Insurance ;

o   Mutualité de l'armée de l'air (MUTAV);

o   Stane insurance;

o   Blue insurance ;

o   Médecins sans Frontières France (MSFF) ;

o   Médecins sans Frontières Belgium (MSFB) ;

o   Qatar Charity;

o   Gras Savoye.

The CHME has signed service agreements with the above-mentioned structures to provide medical care for their sick staff and/or third-party payers.

c-   Foreign partners

As a humanitarian organization, the CHME has developed partnerships with outside organizations and individuals to treat certain pathologies that are difficult to treat in Mali.

The hospital's main partners are :

o   Fondation Luxembourgeoise Raoul Follereau (historical partner) ;

o   Center Hospitalier du Luxembourg (historical partner) ;

o   Chain of Hope ;

o   Terre des hommes ;

o   Principality of Monaco ;

o   SHARE Association;

o   PROBITAS Foundation (Spain) ;

o   CHU - La Rabta, Tunis.

1-2.6 Administrative management

With a current hospitalization capacity of 129 beds, the CHME employs 321 staff in all categories.

These agents are distributed as follows: (see Tables I and II).

Staff	Number
Medical specialists	53
Pharmacists	02
General practitioners	08
Medical assistants	34
Senior technicians	45
Midwives	20
Health technician	49
Obstetric nurses	13
Nursing assistants	18
Administration	57
Social Assistant	03
Maintenance	07
Support staff	10
ARCAD	02
Total	**321**

Ophthalmology department :

-Infrastructure :

- A large consultation room
- Two (2) additional examination rooms
- An optical room
- A toilet in the consultation room

-Human resources :

The staff is composed of 12 agents distributed as follows:

- Four (4) ophthalmologists

- Two (2) medical assistants

- Three (3) optometrists

- One (1) optical space manager

- Two (2) PhD students

Nephrology and hemodialysis department

-Infrastructure :

- A consulting room with a toilet;

- An office for the major, which also serves as an equipment storage area;

- Nurses' room;

- A KT room for dialysis patients;

- A water treatment room;

- A large room containing eight (8) dialysis machines;

- A VIP room containing two (2) dialysis machines;

- Two (2) toilets for patients;

- Two (2) staff toilets;

- A toilet for the doctors in the consulting room;

-Human resources :

The staff is composed of 11 agents distributed as follows:

- Two (2) nephrologists

- Four (4) senior health technicians

- Three (3) health technicians

- Two (2) PhD students

2- Study period :

Our study took place from November 14 to December 14, 2022.

3- Type of study

We conducted a cross-sectional study of hemodialysis patients regularly followed at CHME Le Luxembourg.

4- Study population

The study population consisted of all patients aged 15 and over under regular hemodialysis care and who underwent a complete ophthalmological examination.

5- Sampling

We calculated the sample size using SCHWARTZ's formula $n = z^2.p.\ q/i^2$.

n = sample size

z = confidence level according to the normal distribution (reduced deviation z = 1.96)

p = estimated proportion of the population with the characteristic (frequency = 14 ,8% so p = 0 ,148) [23]

q = 1 -p (q= 1-0 ,148= 0.852)

i= desired precision (we took 10% precision for our study) $n = (1.96)^2 \times 0.148 \times 0.852/ (0.10)^2$

n = 48.44 or 48 Patients

6- Inclusion criteria

All patients over 15 years of age and regularly monitored for hemodialysis, and consenting to the study, were included in the study.

7- Non-inclusion criteria

All hemodialysis patients who did not consent to the study and incomplete records.

8- Support and data collection techniques

In nephrology, data were collected from the patient's medical record and CINZA software, after obtaining consent. The same patients were seen in ophthalmology for a complete examination. A survey form was created to collect all the information required to meet the objectives of our study.

Studied variables :

- Socio-demographic parameters (age, gender, residence, occupation, etc.)

- History of the disease (medical and surgical history, types of renal failure, date of start of dialysis)

- Biological data (Urea, Creatininemia, Hemoglobins, Kalemia, Vitamin D, Calcemia, Platelets, White blood cells, CRP, POu, Natremia, Bicarbonatemia, Albumin, Protidemia, Hepatitis B, Hepatitis C, HIV, TPHA / VDRL)

- The ophthalmological examination :

- Questioning (reason for consultation, general and ophthalmological history)

- External review

- Visual acuity

- Schirmer test (systematic)

Normal	Slight	Moderate	Severe
$\geq$ 15mm	14-9 mm	8-5 mm	$\leq$ 5mm

- Eye tone

- The anterior segment

o The cornea

o La Conjonctive

o La Pupille

o The anterior chamber

o Le Cristallin

- Posterior segment (after dilation with mydriaticum collyre)

o The glass

o Retina (papilla, macula, veins, arteries)

- Complementary examination according to the hypothesis of diagnosis :

o Visual fields

o Pachymetry

o Photo papille

o   AGF

o   OCT

9- data entry and analysis :

Data entry and analysis were carried out using SPSS software.

20.0 and KII2 tcst , filc threshold with 0.05 , results were written using Microsoft Word office 2010

10-   Ethical and deontological considerations

Cases were included with their verbal consent after being informed of the questionnaire's content. The information collected was kept confidential.

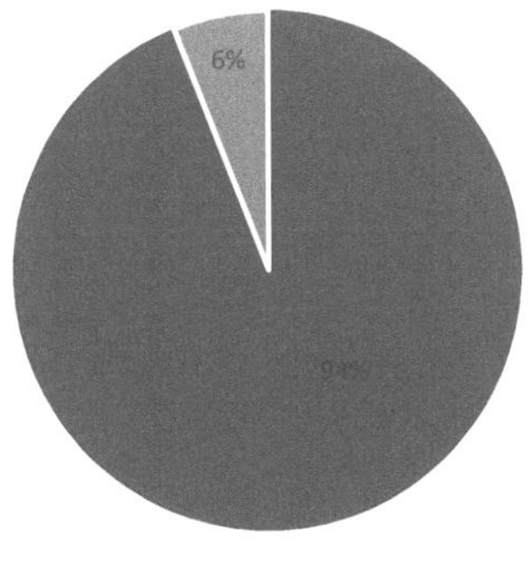

Figure 8: Frequency of ocular complications

During our study, 268 patients were seen in nephrology consultations, including 50 hemodialysis patients. Of these 50 patients, 47 developed an ocular complication, representing a 94% incidence of ocular complications in hemodialysis patients.

2- **Socio-demographic characteristics Table III: Age distribution**

Age range	Workforce	%
< 20 years	4	8
[20-40]	11	22
[41-60]	**28**	**56**
>60 years	7	14
Total	50	100

The 41-60 age group accounted for 56%. The mean age of patients was 47 years, with extremes of 15 and 77 years.

Gender

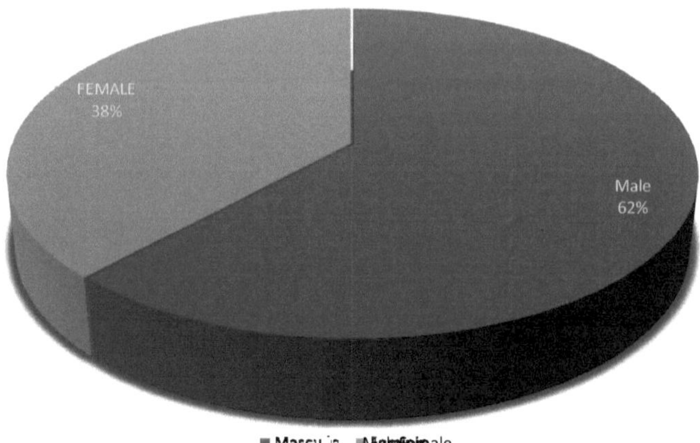

Figure 9: Distribution of patients by gender

Males accounted for 62%, with a sex ratio of 1.6.

Table IV: Breakdown of patients by origin

Communes	Workforce	%	
Commune I	5	10	
Commune II	1		2
Commune III	3		6
Commune I V	**15**	**30**	
Commune V	7	14	
Commune VI	10	20	
Outside communes	9	18	
Total	50	100	

Commune IV was home to 30% of our patients.

Table V: Breakdown of patients by profession

Profession	Workforce		%
Housekeeper	**17**	**34**	
Retailer	9	18	
Cultivator	4		8
Manager	4		8
Student	3		6
Worker	3		6
Driver	2		4
Geological engineer	2		4
Computer scientist	1		2
Teacher	3		6
Military	2		4
Total	50	100	

Housewives accounted for 34% of our patients.

3- Clinical aspects

Nephrological data

Table VI: Distribution of patients by history

History	Workforce		%
Hypertension	**32**	**64**	
Diabetes	1		2
Hypertension +diabetes	13	26	
No antecedents	4		8
TOTAL	50	100	

Hypertension accounted for 64% of the antecedents.

Table VII: Distribution of patients according to initial kidney disease

Initial nephropathy	Workforce	%	
Vascular CKD	**25**	**50**	
Glomerular CKD	21	42	
Functional IRA	4		8
Total	50	100	

Vascular nephropathy accounted for 25 cases or 50% of our patients.

Table VIII: Distribution of patients according to blood calcium levels

Calcemia	Workforce	%
Normal	**26**	**52**
Hypercalcemia	11	22
Hypocalcemia	13	26
Total	50	100

Calcemia levels were normal in 52% of our patients.

Table IX: Distribution of patients by phosphorus level

Phosphoremia	Workforce	%
Normal	15	30
Hyperphosphatemia	**22**	**44**
Hypophosphatemia	13	26
Total	50	100

Hyperphosphatemia was found in 44% of our patients.

Table X: Distribution of patients by severity of hemoglobin level

Hemoglobin level	Workforce	%
<6g	6	12
[6 to 8g]	8	16
[9 to 10g]	**23**	**46**
[11 à 12]	7	14
>to 12g	6	12
Total	50	100

Hemoglobin levels of [9 to 10g] were found in 46% of our patients.

Table X: Distribution of patients by dialysis indication

Indication	Workforce	%
Uremic syndrome	**35**	**70**
Severe acidosis	10	20
OAP	3	6
Hyperkalemia	2	4
Total	50	100

Uremic syndrome was present in 70% of our patients.

Table XI: Distribution of patients by dialysis duration

Duration	Workforce	%
<12 months	**39**	**78**
12 to 24 months	4	8
>24 months	7	14
Total	50	100

The number of patients with a dialysis duration of less than 12 months was 39

(78%). The average duration of dialysis was 8.26 months.

Ophthalmological data :

Table XIII: Distribution of patients according to distance visual acuity (WHO)

Acuity visual	Right eye		Left eye	
	Workforce	%	Workforce	%
$\geq 3/10$	34	68	37	74
[1/10 à 3/10[	8	16	4	8
< 1/10	8	**16**	9	**18**
Total	50	100	50	100

Blindness (AVL< 1/10) was found in 16% of our patients in the right eye and 18% in the left eye.

Table XII: Distribution of patients by intraocular pressure (IOP)

PIO	Right eye		Left eye	
	Workforce	%	Workforce	%
Normal	**46**	**92**	**45**	**90**
Hypertonia	3	6	3	6
Hypotonia	1	2	2	4
Total	50	100	50	100

Intraocular pressure was normal in 92% of our right-eye patients and 90% of our left-eye patients.

TableXV : Distribution of patients according to ophthalmological functional signs

Functional signs	Workforce		%
Yes	**46**	**92**	
No	4		8
Total	50	100	

Functional signs were present in 92% of cases.

Table XIII :   **Distribution   of patients according to ophthalmological functional signs**

Functional signs	Workforce	%
C.E. sensation	**16**	**34,8**
Redness	8	17,4
Tearing	8	17,4
Photophobia	7	15,2
Itching	4	8,7
Swelling of the eyelid	2	4,3
Burning sensation	1	2,2
Total	46	100

The C.E. (strange body) sensation was 34.8% in our study.

Table XIV: Distribution of patients according to dry eyes

Dry eyes	Workforce	Percentage
Yes No Total	**29**	**58**
	21	42
	50	100

Dry eyes were present in 29 cases, i.e. 58% of our patients.

Table XVIII: Distribution of patients according to anterior segment involvement

Anterior segment	Right eye		Left eye	
	Workforce	%	Workforce	%
Lens opacity	**17**	**34**	**17**	**34**
Pterygium	7	14	8	18
Pseudophaque	2	4	2	4
Hyperemia	4	8	3	6
Conjunctival calcification	4	8	3	6
Normal	16	32	17	34
Total	50	100	50	100

Lens opacity was found in 17 cases (34%) in the right and left eyes of our patients with anterior segment disease.

Table XV: Distribution of patients according to posterior segment involvement

Posterior segment	Right eye		Left eye	
	Workforce	%	Workforce	%
Papillary Excavation	2	4	2	4
Papillary pallor	1	2	1	2
Cottony nodule	**12**	**24**	12	**24**
Exudate	6	12	6	12
Cottony nodule +Exudate	5	10	5	10

Papilloedema	2	4	2	4
Macular scarring	1	2	2	4
Macula term Normal	1	2	1	2
	20	40	20	40
Total	50	100	50	100

Cottony nodules were present in 24% of our patients.

Table XX: Distribution of patients according to ocular complications

Ocular complications	Workforce	%
Hypertensive retinopathy	**20**	**40**
Diabetic retinopathy	7	14
Ametropia	6	12
Cataracts	4	8
Pterygium	3	6
Conjunctival calcification	1	2
Optic Neuropathy	1	2
Glaucoma	1	2
HTO	2	4
Conjunctivitis Normal	2	4
	3	6
Total	50	100

Hypertensive retinopathy was found in 40% of our patients.

4- Analytical study

Table XVI: Ocular complications a s a function of vascular chronic renal failure

Ocular complications	Vascular CKD				Total	
	Yes		No			
	Number % of		Number % of total		Workforce	%
Hypertensive retinopathy	**11**	**44**	9	36	20	40
Diabetic retinopathy	0	0	7	28	7	14
Ametropia	5	20	1	4	6	12
Cataracts	3	12	1	4	4	8
Pterygium / Pterygoid	2	8	1	4	3	6
Conjunctival calcification	1	4	0	0	1	2
Optic Neuropathy	0	0	1	4	1	2
Glaucoma	0	0	1	4	1	2
Normal Ophthalmology Exam	1	4	2	8	3	4
Ocular hypertension (HTO)	2	8	0	0	2	4
Conjunctivitis	0	0	2	4	2	2
Total	25	100	25	100	50	100

Hypertensive retinopathy accounted for 44% of vascular chronic renal failure, with a statistically significant difference (P= 0.047 ; Chi2 :18.533).

Table XVIII: Ocular complications as a function of chronic glomerular renal failure

Ocular complications	Glomerular CKD				Total	
	Yes		No			
	Number	% of total		% of	Number	Workforce %
Hypertensive retinopathy	6	35,3	14	42,4	20	40
Diabetic retinopathy	**7**	**41,1**	0	0	7	14
Ametropia	1	5,9	5	15,1	6	12
Cataracts	0	0	4	12,1	4	8
Pterygium / Pterygoid	1	5,9	2	6,1	3	6
Conjunctival calcification	0	0	1	3	1	2
Optic Neuropathy	0	0	1	3	1	2
Glaucoma	1	5,9	0	0	1	2
Ophthalmology examination Normal	1	5,9	2	6,1	3	4
Ocular hypertension (HTO)	0	0	2	6,1	2	4
Conjunctivitis	0	0	2	6,1	2	2
Total	17	100	33	100	50	100

Diabetic retinopathy accounted for 41.1% of glomerular chronic kidney disease, with a statistically significant difference (P= 0.017; Chi2: 21.628).

VI- COMMENTS AND DISCUSSIONS

1- Socio-demographic data :

-Frequency :

In our study, we collected 50 haemodialysis patients out of 268 consultations during the study period. Of these patients, 47 developed ocular complications, a frequency of 94%. This result is similar to those of A. Guennoun et al [33], who found a 100% frequency of ocular complications.

-Age :

The 41-60 age group accounted for 56% of cases, and the mean age of our patients was 47, with extremes ranging from 15 to 77 years. This result is similar to that of I. KARIMI et al [21] who found a mean age of 47+/- 13 years. Diallo.S et al [9] found 41% in the same age bracket, with an average age of 48. Our results differ from those of S. Chiguer et al [7], who found an average age of 41+/-10 years. This difference may be explained by the fact that our sample size is larger than his: 50 hemodialyses versus 26.

-Gender :

Male sex accounted for 62% of cases, with a sex ratio of 1.6. This result concurs with those of S. chiguer et al and Diallo. S et al, who found 57% and 59% respectively [7, 9]. On the other hand, S.R. Ebana Mvogo et al [8] showed a female predominance with 54.3% of cases and a sex ratio of 0.84. This male predominance could be explained by the fact that men are more exposed to cardiovascular risk factors.

-Antecedent :

Hypertension accounted for 64% of cases in our study. KOUASSI FX et al [22] found the same to be true in 65% of cases. I. KARIMI et al [21] found 51.2%. This could be explained by the fact that arterial hypertension is one of the main causes of chronic kidney disease.

-Profession:

In our study, housewives accounted for 34%, followed by shopkeepers with 18%. This result was slightly higher than that of Diallo. S et al [9] who found that 25% were housewives.

2- Nephrological data :

-Duration of dialysis :

Patients with a dialysis duration of less than 12 months accounted for 78% of cases, with an average dialysis duration of 8.26 months. This result differs from those of Diallo. S et al [9] found a frequency of 46.88% of patients with dialysis durations of less than 12 months and an average duration of 3.5 years. This difference could be explained by the study's patient recruitment criteria.

-Initial nephropathy :

In our study, vascular nephropathy represented 50%, followed by glomerular nephropathy 42%. This result is similar to those of Nawal.K et al [2], who found vascular nephropathy at 51.2%, followed by glomerular nephropathy at 30.3%. This could be due to the fact that hypertension represented 64% of the antecedents in our patients, and is the leading cause of CKD, followed by diabetes.

-disorders of phosphocalcic metabolism :

Calcemia was normal in 52% of our patients and hyperphosphatemia in 44%. Our results are similar to those of Diallo. S et al [9] found normal calcemia and hyperphosphatemia in 53% and 50% of cases respectively. This disorder could be explained by the onset of chronic renal failure.

3- Ophthalmological data :

-functional signs :

Foreign body sensation was the functional sign in 32% of cases, followed by lacrimation (16%) and redness (16%). This could be explained by the fact that, in our study, more than half of our patients (58%) had a positive schirmer test (dry eye), making the deficit in tear quality secondary to hemodialysis. According to S.R. Eban Mvogo et al [8], hemodialysis reduces blood urea levels, which in turn leads to a considerable reduction in tear urea levels, thereby lowering tear osmolarity.

-Anterior segment damage:

Lens opacities were found in 34% of cases in the right and left eyes. In contrast, Nawal.K et al [1] and I. KARIMI et al [21] found 40% and 22% of cases respectively. This could be explained by phosphocalcic disturbances, age, duration of hemodialysis, long-term corticosteroid therapy for pre-existing nephropathy and oxidative stress in cataract genesis. Dry eyes were found in 58% of our patients, a result similar to those of S.R. Ebana Mvogo et al [8], who found 40% dry eyes. This could be explained by the fact that our patients were adults, and it is therefore possible that the drop in lacrimal osmolarity could lead to dry eyes.

-Posterior segment damage:

Hypertensive retinopathy was 40% followed by 14% diabetic retinopathy in the posterior segment. This result concurs with those of Nawal.K et al.

[2] who found respectively 45% and 24%, and S. chiguer et al [7] who found respectively 23.07% and 11.5%. This could be explained by the fact that arterial hypertension was 64% of the antecedents found in our patients.

VII- Conclusion

Several ocular anomalies may be encountered in dialysis patients. However, we were able to establish the link between hypertensive retinopathy and chronic renal failure of vascular origin (P= 0.047; Chi2 :18.533) diabetic retinopathy and chronic renal failure of glomerular origin (P= 0.017; Chi2 : 21.628), patients with initial nephropathy were more likely to develop ocular complications such as hypertensive and diabetic retinopathy, hence the need for close collaboration between ophthalmologist and nephrologist.

VIII- RECOMMENDATIONS

At the end of this study, we make the following recommendations:

-To the Minister of Health :

✓ Mobilize the resources needed to facilitate ophthalmological and nephrological care and the various complementary examinations for dialysis patients.

✓ Set up hemodialysis centers in the other communes of the Bamako District.

-To Nephrologists:

✓ Systematically refer dialysis patients for ophthalmological consultations in search of ocular complications

-To ophthalmologists:

✓ Rapid diagnosis of all suspected pathologies in hemodialysis patients to ensure better management.

✓ Diagnose and manage ocular complications ihemodialysis patients.

IX- REFERENCES

[1]   **D. L. Radermacher**. "guide pratique d ' hemodialyse "CHU Liège-site NDB-

URGENCES/SAMU 2004 pp. 1-157

[2]   **Nawal K.** Ophthalmological manifestations in chronic hemodialysis patients. Thèse médecine ,Universite mohamed V de Rabat ,2021 , PP.88 http://bib-fmp.um5.ac.ma/opac_fmp/index.php?lvl=author_see&id=31089

[3]   **Neuen BL, et al.** Chronic kidney disease and the global NCD agenda. BMJ Glob Health. 2017. https://www.who.int/news-room/fact- sheets/detail/the-top-10-causes-of-death

[4]   **Coulibaly, M., Samaké, M., Fofana, A. S., Coulibaly, S. B., Sy, S., Yattara, H., Diallo, D., & Fongoro, S.** Determinants of Mortality among Hemodialysis Patients a t Mali Gavardo Hospital in Sébénikoro (Bamako). HEALTH SCIENCES AND DISEASE, .2020.21(6). Retrieved from https://www.hsd-fmsb.org/index.php/hsd/article/view/2029.

[5]   **JALEL T, et al.** Eye and extra renal purification. Tunis Med 2005, 83(10): 617-21.

[6]   **H. Chen, X. Zhang, and X. Shen, "**Ocular changes during hemodialysis in patients with end-stage renal disease," BMC Ophthalmol. vol. 18, no. 1, pp. 1-9, 2018, doi: 10.1186/s12886-018-0885-0.

[7]   **S. Chiguer et al.** "Manifestations ophtalmologiques chez les hémodialysés chroniques," Néphrologie & Thérapeutique, vol. 16, no. 5, pp. 285-286, 2020, doi: 10.1016/j.nephro.2020.07.090.

[8]   **S. R. Ebana Mvogo et al.** "Measurement of lacrimal secretion in chronic hemodialysis patients at Douala General Hospital - Cameroon," J. Fr. Ophthalmol, vol. 42, no. 3, pp. 244-247, 2019, doi: 10.1016/j.jfo.2018.09.009.

[9]   **Diallo S, Sidibe MK, Napo A, Guirou N, Ba K, Conare I , Cissé I , Guindo A, Sahare F, Traore L, Traore J .**Manifestations ophtalmologiques chez les hémodialyses au mali : à propos de 32 cas .SOAO N° 02-2019 pp. 53-

55.

[10]   Dahami Z, M.D.Elamrani, Bibarchi H .anatomie de l'appareil urinaire : (les reins) université CADI AYY ad Marrakech .33pp.

[11 Bowditch A; Bowditch M. Transverse section of an adult kidney. The Anatomy & Physiology App 2007. University of Utah Spencer S. Eccles Health Sciences Library. https://www.visiblebody.com/fr/learn/urinary/urinary-kidney [date:04/01/2023]

[12]   Drs Aussems, Quéromès, Deschamps Lefèvre, Sitbon and Benarous . anatomie-oeil/#systeme-lacrymal . Center Hospitalier National d'Ophtalmologie des Quinze-Vingts and the Fondation ophtalmologique Adolphe de Rothschild https://www.oph78.fr/ophtalmologie/anatomie-oeil/#systeme-lacrymal [date: 04/01/2023].

[13]   Lucien R, Gabriel C, Silvio D. Oeil et Rein université de paris -vol-de-Marne France. Editions Scientifiques et Médicales Elsevir SAS, Paris [21- 453-A-25] https://www.em-consulte.com/article/7768/resume/oeil-et-rein

[14]   Flament J . Storck D . OEil et pathologie générale . Edition Masson , 1997 , Paris, publisher's boards; large in-8, 822 pp.

[15]   Fattorusso V . Ritter O. Vademecum clinique. From diagnosis to treatment. (17th Edition)Masson, 2004. Paris .pp1970.

[16]   Geremi . Retina Image Bank. 2014; Image 16552/16554. © the American Society of Retina Specialists. Electronic document: https://geremi.fr/index.php/2019/01/07/retinopathie-hypertensive-severe/ Last updated: December 31, 2019.

[17]   Antonetti DA, Klein R, Gardner TW. Diabetic retinopathy. N Engl J Med. 2012 societe française d'ophtalmologie; 366(13): 1227-1239. https://www.em-consulte.com/em/SFO/H2018/B9782294756399000005X.html

[18]   Man N K. Fouan M. Jungers P. Hémodialyse de suppléance .Médecine science. Edition Flammarion 2003. Paris.188P

[19]   **Simon P, Kim S, Christophe C , Philippe Le C.** Dialyse rénale, second edition Masson, June 1999. Paris 8. 05; 55: 1823 1830

[20]   **Tomazzoli L., De Natale R, Lupo A, Parolini B.** Visual acuity disturbances in chronic renal failure. Ophthalmologica, 2000 ;214 (6) : 403-405.

[21]   **I. Karimi et al.** "Ophthalmologic manifestations in chronic hemodialysis patients," Nephrology & Therapeutics, vol. 9, no. 5, pp. 290-291, 2013, doi: 10.1016/j.nephro.2013.07.220.

[22]   **Kouassi FX, Koman CE, Boni S , Gbe K, Berete CR , Soumaro M, Sowagnon T, Kra ANS.** Manifestations ophtalmologiques chez les hémodialysés chroniques : à propos de 100 cas au CHU de cocody. SOAO N°01-2017 ,pp. 39-48

[23]   **Ndiaye Sow MN,Wane AM, Ka AM, Dieng M, Ndoye Roth PA, Ba EA, et al.** Les lesions oculaires chez le patient mélanoderme atteint l'insuffisance rénale chronique .Mali médical 2010 ;25(4) :14-20.

[24]   **COULIBALY G,** et al"Prevalence of ocular abnormalities in hemodialysis patients in Ouagadougou, Burkina Faso". Med Afr Noire 2014. 6111 : 557-63.

[25]   **HACHACHE T, Geurgour M , Gonzalez B et al.** Ophthalmological manifestations in dialysis patients. Retrospective study of 81 patients. Nephrology 1996. 17 (2) ; 117-21.

[26]   **Navdeep G, Aditi S, Reddy VS, Sumita S.** An "eye" on chronic kidney disease International Journal of Advances in Case Reporting. 2015; 2 (16): 1037-1040.

[27]   **REGENBOGEN L., COSCAS G. DEBBASCH S.** Eye and kidney. Encycl.
Med. Chir (Paris - France), Ophthalmology, 21-453-A-25,1995 ; 9

[28]   **VIGNANELLI M. STUCCHI C.A.** Conjunctival calcification in patients in chronic hemodialysis. Morphologic, clinical and epidemiologic study. J. Fr. Ophthalmol, 1988; 11(6-7): 483-492

[29]   **MESARIC B.** Systematic examination of pathological changes in the eyes of patients with chronic renal failure. Arch Ophthalmol 1974; 12, 907-16.

[30]   **PAHOR D, et al.** Conjunctival and corneal changes in chronic renal failure patients treated with maintenance hemodialysis. Ophthalmologica, 1995; 209 (1): 6-14.

[31]   **Tomazzoli L, De Natale R, Lupo A, Parolini B.**Visual acuity disturbances in chronic renal failure. Ophthalmologica. 2000; 214(6):403-5.

[32]   **SIDIBE M. et al** . les atteintes ophtalmologiques chez les insuffisants rénaux chroniques a l'hôpital régional de Sikasso (mali) à propos de 52 cas.revue *SOAO* n° 02- 2022, pp. 9-12

[33]   **A. Guennoun et al.** Ophthalmological complications in dialysis patients :about 50 cases. CHU hôpital Ibn Sina, Rabat, Morocco 13 (2017) 265-295

X- **Appendices :**

Inquiry form

I-IDENTIFICATION:CARD   NUMBER :

FILE :	TEL :
FIRST NAME :	NAME :
AGE :	SEX :
PROFESSION :	ADDRESS :

II- BACKGROUND

1- Medical history

Diabetes1 yes   /_/2 no /_/   Rheumatic disorders 1 yes /_/ 2 no /_/ Thyroid disease 1yes /_/ 2 no /_/ Sarcoidosis 1 yes /_/ 2 no /_/ Skin diseases 1 yes /_/ 2 no /_/   neurodermatitis 1yes /_/ 2 no /_/ Acne rosacea 1yes /_/ 2 no /_/   ichthyosis 1 yes /_/ 2 no /_/ Seborrhea 1 yes /_/ 2 no /_/   Malignant diseases 1 yes /_/ 2 no /_/ Infectious diseases 1 yes /_/ 2 no /_/   HTA 1 yes /_/ 2 no /_/ Others..

2- Surgical history

Trigeminal nerve operation 1 yes /_/2   no /_/

Others..

3- Treatment history

Anticholinergics   /_/Antihistamines /_/Antiarrhythmics /_/ Analgesics /_/ Antihypertensives /_/ (beta-blockers, reserpine, thiazide diureticsetc...

)Antidepressants/_/Neuroleptics   /_/Psychotropic   drugs /_/ Estrogens /_/ Cytostatics /_/ Antimigraine drugs /_/ Oral contraceptives /_/ Others...

III-   NEPROLOGY A- IRC

1) Glomerular origin: 1= Yes 2= No

2) Vascular origin: 1=Yes 2=No

3) Tubulo interstitial: 1=Yes 2=No

4) Origin undetermined: 1=Yes 2=No B: IRA (GNRP) :

1   :Gourgerot schogren 1=Yes 2=No

2   :LET 1=Yes 2=No

3   Scleroderma 1=Yes 2=No

4   Good Pasture 1=Yes 2=No

5   Periarteritis Noueuse   1=Yes2=No

6   Wegener's disease 1=Yes   2=No

C-Biological

1. Urea :

2. Creatininemia

3. GFR: 1= Grade I 3= Grade III 5= Grade V 2= Grade II4=   Grade IV

4. Hb = Plq = GB =

5. Calcemia = 10. CRP =

6. POu = 11.Natremie =

7. PTH = 12.Kaliemie =

8. VITD = 13.Bicarbonalemie =

9. Albumin = 14.protein =

D - Infectious

-HVB: 1= Positive 2= Negative

-HVC: 1= Positive 2= Negative

-HIV: 1= Positive 2= Negative

-TPHA VDRL: 1= Positive 2= Negative

E-Hemodialysis

-VA   =1=   FAV2= KTF

-DPS=

-PPID =

-Heparin =

-DD Dialysis =

-Capillary =

-KT/V =

-Dialysat flow =

-Restitution =

Indications for dialysis: 1-Hyperkalemia /_/ 2-Severe acidosis /_/ 3-OAP /_/ 4-Uremic syndrome /_/ 5-Uremic pericarditis /_/ Start date of dialysis :

Duration/Session :

Dialysis rhythm: ½   week2/3 week

IV OPHTHALMOLOGY

1- QUESTIONING :

Redness of the eye   /_/Sensation of EC /_/Sensation   of

dryness /_/ Sensation of burning eyes /_/ Swelling of the eyelids

        /_/Sensitivity to light /_/ Tearing /_/ Epiphora /_/ Sensation of tiredness

/_/ Itching /_/ Sensitivity to tobacco smoke /_/ to air conditioning (to ventilation

in cars) /_/ other environmental influences /_/

2- Schirmer test

	Normal	Slight	Moderate	Severe
	≥ 15mm	14-9 mm	8-5 mm	≤ 5mm
Right eye				
Left eye				

Dry   eyesYes   //No   //

3- the parameters

	Right eye	Left eye
AVL/SC		
AVL/AC		
AVP		
PIO		

4- Explorations

Slit lamp	Right eye	Left eye
Anterior segment		
Posterior segment		
Total		

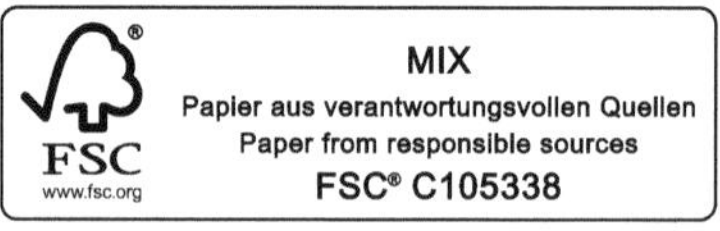

Printed by Books on Demand GmbH, Norderstedt / Germany